Journey Toward Heaven: Entering Eternity

JOURNEY TOWARD HEAVEN: ENTERING ETERNITY

PAM BROWN

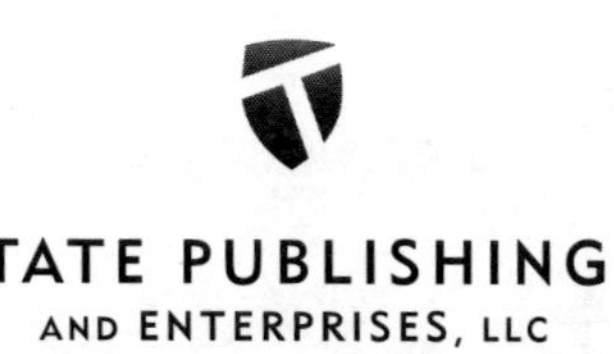

TATE PUBLISHING
AND ENTERPRISES, LLC

Acknowledgments

Writing my first book has been a wonderful journey but would not have been possible without key people walking that journey with me.

To my husband, Mark, who has inspired, prayed, and encouraged me to follow my heart in writing this book. You have given me many helpful insights throughout my first writing journey. You are the love of my life!

To my good friend Sue Lenarz who proofread many manuscripts and offered invaluable suggestions. Thanks, Sue, for your continual prayers, encouragement, and positive support for me.

To Shawna and David Keaton and Greg and Summer Brown, my wonderful grown children, you have loved and enthusiastically motivated me to complete this book.

This book is dedicated to my family, friends, and my grandson, Timothy, who makes my heart melt.

I love you all lots!

Contents

Journey Toward Heaven

Names of the Saved Are Written in Heaven

Notwithstanding in this rejoice not, that the spirits are subject unto you; but rather rejoice, because your names are written in heaven. (Luke 10:20, NASB)

In the Bible, the New Testament book of Luke tells us to be exuberant because those of us who have trusted and believed in Christ have our names written in heaven. God regards us as so important that he writes our names down in a book called the book of life. Once your name is written in the book of life, it will never be erased, blotted out, or marked off; it is written there forever and ever.

Another book was opened, which is the book of life. (Revelations 20:12, NIV)

The Bible speaks of heaven as a place for Christians to live forevermore when they leave this earth and enter eternity. The promise of heaven comforts our hearts and gives us a real hope, a place to contemplate and excitedly look forward to.

When my dad was diagnosed with cancer, the doctors gave him just thirty days to live. Our family went into shock for about a week before we could actually cope with the situation. Death is shocking even though someday we will all have to face it personally. For some reason, none of us believe that death is something we need to think about until we are forced to. My dad actually lived for the next six months. Every year he would always complain about having to paying taxes. "Tax, taxes, taxes" is what he would say each year when April 15 came around. Our family found this amusing and so each year we would tease him about his treaded fate of paying taxes. He was diagnosed in August of 1990 and then passed away (would you believe it?) on tax day, April 15, 1991! Who says God doesn't have a sense of humor!

Coping with a terminal illness is not easy; actually, it is very difficult for an entire family, ours included. We did make the most of every day by searching for something to laugh and smile about. You would be surprised at how creative you can be and at the things that you can come up with when you set your mind on being joyful. Each day became an adventure for all of us. When we had a down day, someone would come up with a crazy story to cheer that person up. We took leisurely walks and actually noticed some things that we had never observed before—the beauty of a rose, the many veins that show in a leaf, how many different types of colors or minerals in a rock. These are things that none of us become aware of unless we take the time to look and study them for a few minutes. Because we live in such a "hurry up" world, often the small wonderful things in nature go unnoticed. When we purposely take a few minutes to look at a flower, we see all the things that make up that flower: petals, leaves, thorns, pollen, stamen, stem, rose hips (seed pods of roses which are edible), etc. Nature is incredible, fascinating, amusing, and reveals just some of what heaven possesses.

I have worked with parents of cancer children for over twenty-five years and have been asked numerous times, "What book would you recommend for us to read to our loved ones who are in their final days on earth?" Families who are faced with watching and caring for a loved one who is very close to death want to comfort them in every way possible. Reading about heaven is comforting and helps families cope with the end of life process. Therefore, I have always recommended reading a children's Bible. A children's Bible has biblical stories that are condensed, complete, and easy to understand and simple to read for all ages. During the last two weeks of my dad's life, our family took turns every day reading Bible stories to him. We read from a children's Bible, and he looked forward each day to one of us reading to him.

Although a children's Bible is fabulous, it doesn't always answer some very probing questions adults and children have about the afterlife. So I have thought over and over again that a book on heaven would encourage the readers and comfort the dying.

Heaven

- Where is it?
- What's it like?
- Who will be there?
- How do I get there?
- Is there a certain place that I will have to find, like a light or tunnel?
- What will I do when I get there?
- How can I be sure that's where I will be?

These are just a few of the questions that I have been asked by adults and children who were on their deathbeds. Questions like those can be a difficult topic for most people to answer. Therefore, I am writing to both the living and to those who are passing from this life as we know it and transitioning to their eternal home in heaven.

This book is dedicated to those we love.

Where Is Heaven's Location? It's "Up"

From heaven the Lord looks down and sees all mankind; from his dwelling place he watches all who live on earth. (Psalm 33:13–14, NIV)

This is what the Lord says: Heaven is my throne and the earth is my footstool. (Isaiah 66:1, NIV)

God, when searching mankind, looks down from heaven. We as people, when seeking God, always look up toward the sky. When Stephen was martyred, he looked up toward heaven and saw the glory of heaven, and Jesus standing in honor at God's right hand. (Acts 7:56)

Elijah was taken *up* to heaven by a whirlwind (2 Kings 2:11). When the disciple John was about to be given a tour of heaven, he was invited to "*come up.*"
Heaven is up

- Above the atmosphere
- Beyond the stratosphere
- Past the exosphere
- Outside of our interplanetary space
- Heaven is up above our solar system

- Farther than the billions of galaxies
- And higher than the trillions of stars in our universe

Mankind is, and has always been, fascinated with the universe with its stars, planets, and galaxies. Hundreds of movies have been produced with the theme of space, different life-forms, and what exists beyond our universe. Scientists have continually been captivated in exploring space to see what they can find that is unusual and never before seen. Throughout time, several new and remarkable galaxies have been revealed. Modern instruments and more powerful telescopes will continue to be invented to go beyond what has already been discovered. Scientists will keep on exploring and probing deeper into the cosmos, always on the lookout for new galaxies, planets, universes, and different life-forms.

Space is thrilling, exhilarating, and will remain a subject that will always captivate the imagination. But I am convinced that we, as mankind, will never discover all the galaxies and universes that exist. I believe that God allows mankind to locate them a little at a time to keep us mesmerized and intrigued by the greatness and vastness of the universe. Experts have said that there are so many stars in the sky that they outnumber the earth's population by one trillion stars to each and every person. Isaiah 40 tells us that God calls each star by name and he keeps a count of them. If God keeps an account of all the stars, how much more does he value us? God loves us so much that he keeps heaven's door open always just waiting for us to knock on it and invite him to be a part of our lives (Revelation 3:20),

> Lift your eyes and look to the heavens: Who created all these? He who brings out the starry host one by one, and calls them each by name. Because of his great power and mighty strength, not one of them is missing. (Isaiah 40:26, NIV)

The Bible tells us over and over again that heaven is *up*. No matter what continent you are on, what time zone you are in, or wherever you are on earth, God is *up*. God says He is all around us, He's everywhere, and He is not limited by space or any realm. What mankind struggles with is the notion that there must be more to space than just space. God, on the other hand, states that He is the creator of mankind, the cosmos, and the heavens. God is the maker of everything that man knows and doesn't know.

> The heavens declare the glory of God; the skies proclaim the work of his hands. (Psalms 19:1, NIV)

> Acknowledge and take to heart this day that the LORD is God in heaven above and on the earth below. There is no other. (Deuteronomy 4:39, NIV)

There will be a time when those who are alive on the earth will see the clouds part and Christ standing at the right hand of God. Those who have believed in Christ as their savior will be called *up* to join Him (1 Thessalonians 4:17). We can be assured that heaven is *up*; how far *up*, we don't know. We will just have to wait until it's our time to pass from earth into eternity to see heaven for ourselves.

> And our God fills both the whole of heaven and earth. (Jeremiah 23:24, NIV)

What Is It Like?

Often heaven is thought of as having little cherublike beings floating on clouds presided over by a God sporting a long white beard, standing with staff in hand, high on a mountaintop, surrounded by big puffy white clouds.

But the Bible describes heaven as so much more than that. The beauty is indescribable with rivers, trees, animals, gardens, fruit, gold, jewels, and spectacular bright lights.

> The wall was made of jasper, and the city of pure gold, as pure as glass. The foundations of the city walls were decorated with every kind of precious stone. (Revelation 21:18, NIV)

Heaven is the dwelling place of God. It's a place where God lives and where God is worshipped. We are told by the disciple Matthew that heaven is like a treasure hidden in a field. It's a place of flawlessness, happiness, and contentment. No agony, no sorrow, no grief, no conflicts, and God will wipe every tear from our eyes.

We are assured there will be

• No more death	• No troubles
• No suffering	• No disabilities
• No pain	• No sickness
• No mortgage	• No hurting
• No rent	• No enemies
• No violence	• No darkness
• No danger	• No night
• No fear	• No sea
• No guilt	• No sun or moon
• No destruction	• And that gravity will be absent or radically reduced
• No wars	

NO DEATH

> He will wipe away every tear from their eyes;
> and there will no longer be any death; there will
> no longer be any mourning, or crying, or pain.
> (Revelation 21:4, NASU)

Forever death is abolished, wiped away, vanquished, never to resurface. Death and dying—we are constantly surrounded by it every single day. We are reminded about the circle of life when we watch the seasons change throughout the year—fall, winter, spring, and summer. Leaves on a tree start the dying process in the fall; they change colors and then fall off the trees to crumple and break into little pieces on the ground. Then, in the spring, new leaves will bud, fruit will start to form, and the life-growing process begins again. It's difficult to imagine a world without the possibility of dying. But there is no such thing in heaven; we will never have to think about dying or leaving our loved ones again.

> For everything there is a season, and a time for very purpose under heaven. (Ecclesiastes 3:1, ASV)

NO SUFFERING

There is so much suffering in the world today—disease, hunger, crime, torture, and the list goes on and on. Imagine walking on a street that has no inkling of crime distress or death. You can walk freely just concentrating on the beauty that surrounds you—mountains that are snowcapped, vast green meadows with birds singing, and ponds of crystal clear water. What awesome calm and peaceful thoughts that come to mind, and suffering is nowhere in your thoughts!

NO SEA, NO OCEANS!

> Then I saw a new heaven and a new earth, for the first heaven and the first earth had passed away, and there was no longer any sea. (Revelation 21:1, NIV)

I love to sit on the sand of a beach. For me, sitting there and looking at the water is very calming. The sound of the waves crashing and the smell of the seawater spray blowing over my face is very soothing. There I can imagine the greatness of God by sitting quietly on the sand, looking and listening to the sounds, and experiencing all the smells of ocean. The sea holds amazing creatures and fascinating plant life. When I think of the sea, I think of dolphins, whales, seashells, sea creatures, and the most beautiful aqua-green water. However, the sea has a particularly frightening and dark side as well

When snorkeling in Hawaii one summer, I became so engrossed in following some very unique fish that I forgot about everything else in the world. The beauty of the fish and plant life were the only things that had my mind and attention. Then, all of a sudden, everything changed, and I could not see the bottom of the ocean floor, instantly there was only darkness all around me. Darkness is extremely terrifying, especially in the ocean. It was then that I looked up to find myself in very deep water far from the shore. Panic began to set in, my heart began to beat a little louder, and my thoughts went immediately to visions of some very large dangerous fish that could be close by me. Hawaii is known to have some of the bigger, more aggressive sharks in the world, so of course, that is what my mind began to picture swimming below me, though I couldn't see them. Darkness is the absence of light, it's blackness with obscurity, and very gloomy. Darkness holds an immense grip on us because we can't see what's around us, and our minds picture very chilling things lurking in the shadows. After praying to calm myself down, and taking in a few deep breaths to help me think straight, I began my trek back to shallow water. After several long, agonizing minutes of swimming and trying to stay calm, I did make it back to shore and vowed never to let that happen again.

After contemplating a world with no sea, I began to realize that the oceans, no matter how intriguing they are, hold some of the most frightening things on earth. The dark depths of the sea and the creatures they contain are chilling, intimidating, poisonous, dangerous, and daunting. Death is often related to the dark depths of the sea and with good reason. The seas and oceans of the world have and continue to claim the lives of hundreds of people every year. Heaven will not contain evil in any form because Satan is banished, and all that is evil and dark will be banished with him, gone forevermore. Nothing impure will ever enter into heaven nor will anyone who does wickedness, shameful, or deceitful acts. The only people in heaven will be those whose names are written down in Christ's book of life. So we will not miss the seas or oceans because God has other things in store for us. Gone is *all darkness*, no more scary things that move in the night. Gone is *all evil* and all the things associated with evil.

We will live in a world without darkness or wickedness of any sort. Only goodness and light will surround us all day, every day. We will be safe and worry free. What an awesome promise God has given us!

There Will Be No Sun or Moon in Heaven

> The city does not need the sun or the moon to shine
> on it, for the glory of God gives it light, and the
> Lamb is its lamp. (Revelation 21:23–24, NIV)

The moon's gravitational influence produces the oceans' tides every day. Tides are the rise and fall of sea levels caused by the combined effects of the gravitational forces exerted by the moon and the sun and the rotation of the earth. There won't be "time" as we know it today because there is no night in heaven, only light. Therefore, there is no need of a moon to produce a gravitational pull to change the tides or a sun to produce light. The lack of the sun's brightness is not a problem; the Bible tells us that the glory of God Himself is so brilliant that it will provide all the illumination needed. Heaven is more beautiful than any of us can envision, more breathtaking than anything that has ever been seen by human eyes.

> You will go out in joy and be led forth in peace; the
> mountains and hills will burst into song before you,
> and all the trees of the field will clap their hands.
> (Isaiah 55:12, NIV)

Imagine waving fields of green grass, breathtaking snowcapped mountains, lake water so clear and motionless it looks like a mirror reflecting everything on its still, calm surface that surrounds it. Stars shining in the sky where there is no darkness, yet they are clearly seen. Trees that reach up as high as we can see with bright green leaves on every branch, they seem so cheerful and content standing tall and straight. In heaven, everything as we know it now will be changed to that which is far beyond our imaginations. A brand-new type of day awaits us in heaven.

> No longer will you need the sun or moon to give you light, for the Lord your God will be your everlasting light, and he will be your glory. Your sun shall never set; the moon shall not go down-for the Lord will be your everlasting light; your days of mourning all will end. (Isaiah 60:19–21, TLB)

> There will be no more night. They will not need the light of a lamp or the light of the sun, for the Lord God will give them light. And they will reign forever and ever. (Revelation 22:5, NIV)

GUILT

Guilt is debilitating and a constant reminder of what we should have done instead of what we did. God promises total forgiveness once we ask Him. Jesus spoke many times on forgiveness. In the Sermon on the Mount in Matthew, Jesus spoke about "Blessed are the merciful for they will be shown mercy." He told us to forgive others seventy times seven, to love our enemies…the list is endless throughout the New Testament regarding Jesus's teachings on forgiving others.

Therefore, there is now no condemnation for those who are in Christ Jesus. (Romans 8:1, NIV)

The Lord is good, a refuge in times of trouble. He cares for those who trust in him. (Nahum 1:7, NIV)

If we confess our sins, he is faithful and just and will forgive us our sins and purify us from all unrighteousness. (1 John 1:9–10, NIV)

Once we truly understand and grasp that God has really forgiven us, we are faced with the task of forgiving ourselves or forgiving someone else. *We don't forgive a person who has wronged or hurt us for their sake. We forgive them in our heart— for our sake.* The resentment, anger, and *making-them-pay* attitude will consume us if we don't let our mind and heart come to peace about a situation. We have to let that wrong go for our own well-being and health, remembering that God is our advocate, and He will take revenge for us. Leave it in God's hands for God says, "Vengeance is mine."

The Lord is a jealous and avenging God; the Lord takes vengeance and is filled with wrath. The Lord takes vengeance on his foes and maintains his wrath against his enemies. The Lord is slow to anger and great in power; the Lord will not leave the guilty unpunished. (Nahum 1:2–3, NIV)

Heaven Described

The apostle John describes heaven as immeasurable, expansive, and glorious. God is seated in the center of this amazing, glittering, dazzling array of sparkling jewels. The streets are made of gold, gold so bright and brilliant that it appears as if transparent (Revelation 10:1).

There will be

- Never-ending beauty
- Glorious amazement
- Brilliant light
- True fellowship
- Complete forgiveness
- Oodles of laughter
- Joy beyond comparison
- Perfect peace
- Total protection
- Pure kindness
- Absolute love
- Grace and mercy
- We will receive a new body
- And we'll have the astounding *security* of being with God forever

Heaven is the flawlessness of beauty in every sense. We will be able to *feel* the wonder and *love* of everything around us, nothing ugly will we ever see or experience again.

Who Resides There?

Jesus answered, "I am the way and the truth and the life. No one comes to the Father except through me." (John 14:6, NIV)

God sits in the center of the New Jerusalem. The New Jerusalem is the Holy City of God which is created for those who of us who have made a prior reservation.

And the one who sat there had the appearance of jasper and carnelian. A rainbow, resembling an emerald, encircled the throne. (Revelation 4:3, NIV)

The apostle John in the book of Revelation was invited *up* to enter God's place of residence. John describes what he saw there; God is seated in the very center of heaven on an enormous throne. Encircling God were twenty-four other thrones, and on them sat twenty-four elders of the earth. The elders were dressed in white and wore gold crowns on their heads. From the center of the circle where God is seated there were flashes of lightning, rumblings, and peals of thunder. Lightning, rumblings, and thunder are expressive of God's holiness, righteousness, and power.

The clouds poured down water, the skies resounded with thunder; your arrows flashed back and forth.

Your thunder was heard in the whirlwind, your lightning lit up the world; the earth trembled and quaked. (Psalms 77:17–18, NIV)

The LORD will roar from Zion and thunder from Jerusalem; the earth and the sky will tremble. (Joel 3:16, NIV)

There's a magnificent enormous rainbow that encircles the throne of God. When we see a rainbow today, we see what appears as an arc of a rainbow that touches the ground on both sides. This rainbow that is described in heaven is a complete circle, not a portion of an arc or half of a circle. In heaven, all things are completed and finished, nothing is left unfinished. The rainbow today reminds us of God's covenant with Noah, a symbol of God's promise that He would never again destroy the earth with a flood. Genesis 9:13 tells us that God's covenant was given to Noah but intended for all of His creation, which includes us. Recently while on a flight, we saw a bright, beautiful rainbow outside of our airplane window. We were fifteen thousand feet in the air and there it was, with clouds intertwined all around the arc as it reached high into the atmosphere; it was totally mesmerizing. God's reminding and showing his love for us.

Surrounding the throne were twenty-four other thrones, and seated on them were twenty-four elders. They were dressed in white and had crowns of gold on their head. From the throne came flashes of lightning, rumblings and peals of thunder. (Revelation 4:4–5, NIV)

There are angelic beings, elders, the twelve apostles, and a great assembly of the redeemed of the earth. These great assemblies of the redeemed are all the people gathered from every nation, tribe, and peoples. The society of heaven is select; it's for those who've trusted in Christ while here on earth prior to death.

We will be an exalted family member in heaven, one member of a very huge family. Not the typical dysfunctional family we now know, but a family that will be at peace with one another. We will have a family that really cares and loves one another immeasurably.

But now he has reconciled you by Christ's physical body through death to present you holy in his sight, without blemish and free from accusation. (Colossians 1:22, NIV)

The "noes" of heaven

• No anger	• No suspicion
• No animosity	• No hostility
• No arguments	• No inferiority
• No arrogance	• No jealousy
• No bitterness	• No pride
• No conceit	• No resentment
• No death	• No self-importance

• No disputes	• No sibling rivalry
• No envy	• No smugness
• No fear	• No superiority
• No hatred	

Those will be replaced with

• Blamelessness	• Hope
• Calmness	• Humility
• Contentment	• Joy
• Delight	• Kindness
• Excellence	• Life
• Faith	• Peace
• Fascination	• Righteousness
• Gentleness	• Serenity
• Goodness	• Tranquility
• Happiness	• Trust
• Harmony	• Virtue
• Honesty	• Wonder
• Honor	• And a genuine love for one another. Marvelous!

God promises that those who believe in their heart and confess with their mouth that Jesus is Lord will have a place in heaven reserved just for them. Their reservations are made and their names written down in the book of life.

That if you confess with your mouth, "Jesus is Lord," and believe in your heart that God raised him from the dead, you will be saved. For it is with your heart that you believe and are justified, and it is with your mouth that you confess and are saved. (Romans 10:9–11, NIV)

Now we know that if the earthly tent we live in is destroyed, we have a building from God, an eternal house in heaven, not built by human hands. (2 Corinthians 5:1, NIV)

Heaven is real, it's stable, secure, permanent, and will be our eternal home. Heaven has many houses, palaces, and mansions; it contains our never-ending residence. A home without fences or walls, and the most important item in this residence is not the dwelling itself but the people that reside in it—*you and I.*

You are extremely important to God, you are loved by and measured as priceless to Him. Doesn't that make you feel so special that God considers you to be of the utmost value regardless of your past? Once you ask God for forgiveness, all is forgiven and forgotten; your new life begins immediately. Your slate has been wiped clean for He has cast your sins as far as the east is from the west. What is so fascinating about that statement is that the east and west never meet, so your sin is forever forgotten by God, never to be remembered again. You now have a new beginning, and your reservation in heaven is made with your name written in the book of life.

> He has removed our sins as far away from us as the east is from the west. (Psalms 103:12–13, TLB)

> If we claim to be without sin, we deceive ourselves and the truth is not in us. If we confess our sins, he is faithful and just and will forgive us our sins and purify us from all unrighteousness. (1 John 1:8–9, NIV)

> For I will forgive their wickedness and will remember their sins no more. (Hebrew 8:12, NIV)

> Therefore, if anyone is in Christ, he is a new creation; the old has gone, the new has come! (2 Corinthians 5:17–18, NIV)

WILL I BE MARRIED?

The Lord God said, "It is not good for the man to be alone. I will make a helper suitable for him." (Genesis 2:18, NIV)

God established marriage for companionship and procreation. There is no need for marriage in heaven because there is no death, no need to have children to populate the earth, and no need for marital companionship. In heaven, we will be surrounded by multitudes of believers, angels, and God; we will never be lonely again.

> Jesus replied, "The people of this age marry and are given in marriage. But those who are considered worthy of taking part in that age and in the resurrection from the dead will neither marry nor be given in marriage, and they can no longer die; for they are like the angels. They are God's children, since they are children of the resurrection." (Luke 20:34–36, NIV)

> After this I looked and there before me was a great multitude that no one could count, from every nation, tribe, people and language, standing before the throne and in front of the Lamb. (Revelation 7:9, NIV)

But we will recognize each other. In the garden of Gethsemane, the disciples recognized Elijah and Moses. Yet these two guys had died over seven hundred years prior. The disciples could no way have ever met Elijah or Moses, yet they knew who they were. We may not be married, but we are comforted to know that we will recognize and love our spouses.

> When the dead rise, they will neither marry nor be given in marriage; they will be like the angels in heaven. (Mark 12:25, NIV)

WILL I KNOW ANYONE?

- God lives there,
- Christ lives there,
- The Redeemed who have already passed away live there
- And angels live there

> For by him all things were created: things in heaven and on earth, visible and invisible, whether thrones or powers or rulers or authorities; all things were created by him and for him. (Colossians 1:16, NIV)

We have been created for love, friendship, and a binding union with our friends. I have several loved ones already in heaven, my parents, a son, several grandchildren, family members, and friends. Because I have people that I love already walking the streets of gold in heaven, heaven doesn't seem so foreign and frightening but inviting and familiar. When we know that we will be surrounded by God and our loved ones, we begin to actually look forward to seeing them again. Our fear starts to dissipate when we are assured that death is not the end but that God loves us and desires for us to live in such a wonderful place with Him.

God never designed us to be alone, by ourselves, or to be solitary. God has called us as Christians to practice the "one anothers."

Greet One Another
Greet one another with a kiss of love. (1 Peter 5:14, NIV)

Teach One Another
I myself am convinced, my brothers, that you yourselves are full of goodness, complete in knowledge and competent to instruct one another. (Romans 15:14, NIV)

Be Devoted to One Another
Be devoted to one another in brotherly love. (Romans 12:10a, NIV)

Be Compassionate to One Another
This is what the LORD Almighty says: Administer true justice; show mercy and compassion to one another. (Zechariah 7:9, NIV)

Accept One Another
Therefore, accept one another, just as Christ also accepted us to the glory of God. (Romans 15:7, NASU)

Fellowship With One Another
Speak to one another with psalms, hymns and spiritual songs. (Ephesians 5:19, NIV)

Be Kind to One Another

Be kind and compassionate to one another. (Ephesians 4:32, NIV)

Love one another as brothers, and be kind and humble with one another. (1 Peter 3:8b, TEV)

Serve One Another

Rather, serve one another in love. (Galatians 5:13, NIV)

Be Patient to One Another

Be completely humble and gentle; be patient, bearing with one another in love. (Ephesians 4:2, NIV)

Help One Another

And we urge you, brothers, warn those who are idle, encourage the timid, help the weak. (1 Thessalonians 5:14, NIV)

Be Truthful to One Another

These are the things which you should do: speak the truth to one another. (Zechariah 8:16, NASU)

You shall not steal, nor deal falsely, nor lie to one another. (Leviticus 19:11, NASU)

Show Mercy to One Another

Blessed are the merciful, for they will be shown mercy. (Matthew 5:7, NIV)

Honor One Another

> *Love one another with brotherly affection as members of one family, giving precedence and showing honor to one another. (Romans 12:10, AMP)*

Be Humble to One Another

> *All of you, clothe yourselves with humility toward one another. (1 Peter 5:5, NIV)*

Forgive One Another

> *Bear with each other and forgive whatever grievances you may have against one another. (Colossians 3:13, NIV)*

Encourage One Another

> *But encourage one another daily, as long as it is called Today. (Hebrews 3:13, NIV)*

> *Therefore encourage one another and build each other up. (1 Thessalonians 5:11, NIV)*

Love One Another

> *A new command I give you: Love one another. (John 13:34, NIV)*

> *And now these three remain: faith, hope and love. But the greatest of these is love. (1 Corinthians 13:13, NIV)*

So of course we will recognize one another; the *"one anothers"* are highly valuable to God.

When we are standing at the graveside of a family member, friend, or someone we love, our heart is truly broken. This cry of our heart is not a delusion; it's very real. We truly, honestly miss those we love. But God reassures us of a joyful and everlasting reunion that awaits us just beyond the grave in our eternal home: heaven. So for now, our soul will miss and yearn for those who have gone before us. But we will continue to hold them close to our hearts until we see them again in heaven.

> Blessed are those who mourn, for they will be comforted. (Matthew 5:4, NIV)

> Love the Lord your God with all your heart and with all your soul and with all your strength and with all your mind; and, "Love your neighbor as yourself." (Luke 10:27, NIV)

Our Body?

They are natural human bodies now, but when they are raised, they will be spiritual bodies. For just as there are natural bodies, so also there are spiritual bodies. (1 Corinthians 15:44, NLT)

But our homeland is in heaven, and we are waiting for our Savior, the Lord Jesus Christ, to come from heaven. By his power to rule all things, he will change our simple bodies and make them like his own glorious body. (Philippians 3:20–21, NCV)

The world today places so much emphasis on having a "beautiful" body. Hair care products, cosmetics, ageless products, health equipment, and weight loss merchandises are billion-dollar-a-year businesses.

Products that guarantee

- less wrinkles
- no gray hair
- gadgets for firming and toning muscles
- more energy
- a thinner body
- smooth skin
- antiaging

- vitamins to live a longer life beautiful, younger-looking skin
- etc., etc., etc.

All of these products promise to make us presentable and acceptable to society and the world. Thankfully, these are things that we will not have to worry about in our future life. We won't have to worry about our wardrobes, being in fashion, or what others may judge us on. The body that we have now is subject to so many things—injury, aging, infection, and death. Our bodies today are designed for this earth; we need air, food, gravity, sunlight, and sleep.

Our new bodies in heaven will be imperishable and free of those boundaries because God will give us new heavenly bodies that will be in top physical condition and perfect in every way. Imagine having a new body that won't be crippled by disease or age. A body that will be able to walk, run, and be free of the worry of pain. We won't have to be concerned about weight, sickness, disabilities, aging, imperfections, or limitations. Our new bodies will be just like God designed them to be—free of death, harm, and anything defective. A new body that is flawless and clothed in righteousness and without sin.

> But you have come to Mount Zion, to the heavenly Jerusalem, the city of the living God. You have come to thousands upon thousands of angels in joyful assembly, to the church of the firstborn, whose

names are written in heaven. You have come to God, the judge of all men, to the spirits of righteous men made perfect. (Hebrews 12:22–23, NIV)

Our Bodies Today
- Are mortal and destined for death
- They are weak and susceptible to disease and time
- They are imperfect and sinful
- They are natural bodies made of flesh and blood

Our New Bodies in Heaven
- Will be imperishable and never to die again
- Will be raised in God's power and glory
- Will be glorified and free of all unrighteousness
- They are a new spiritual body specially designed by God

Our brains won't be limited by illness, IQ, confusion, forgetfulness, culture, tradition, or beliefs. We will have the ability to learn and the capability to understand all that God intended for us to know and learn. The small amount of knowledge that we can acquire now on earth stands in no proportion to the learning capabilities we will possess in heaven. God tells us that what we now know is only in part, but in heaven, we will know all things fully.

Now we see but a poor reflection as in a mirror; then we shall see face to face. Now I know in part;

then I shall know fully, even as I am fully known. (1 Corinthians 13:12, NIV)

God created us for wisdom and for the possession of truth, perfect in its kind. He also made us for holiness, for a complete and final accomplishment over wrongdoing, and for the perfect and secure possession of virtue. Virtue has all the characteristics that God intended for us to have—decency, kindness, moral excellence, goodness, honesty, integrity, righteousness, and honor. All those characteristics will be restored to us when we enter eternity.

But the fruit of the Spirit is love, joy, peace, patience, kindness, goodness, faithfulness, gentleness and self-control. (Galatians 5:22–23a, NIV)

What Will I Do When I Get There?

Some think that the only activity in heaven we will do is to pray and worship God. That thought only brings one word to mind: uninspiring! That can't be the only activities that God has in store for us! It just doesn't give us warm fuzzies to think that all we will have to do every day and all day long is to worship God and maybe take a nap. If that is all that heaven has to offer, most of us wouldn't get too excited about being there. But when reading through the Old Testament, you see a totally different concept about God. God was always directing the Israelite nation to celebrate. So celebrations became a huge part of their culture.

They celebrated

- New harvests
- New moon
- New Year
- First day of the month
- Freedom
- Sabbaths
- Dedication of a child
- Family and friends
- Birthdays
- Faith

Parties were a customary activity of the Israelite nation. Celebrations for religious observances, festivals, banquets, feasts for great family occasions such as a birthday, the weaning of a son and heir, a marriage, the reunion of friends, a burial, and even sheepshearing. Parties were given at every opportunity. Celebrations bring family and friends together, which builds unity and fellowship. We will take part of wonderful and glorious festivities in heaven. We will enjoy and love celebrating a holy, merciful, and gracious God and all that He has given us (Leviticus 23).

They will celebrate your abundant goodness and joyfully sing of your righteousness. (Psalm 145:7, NIV)

A few Bible references:

- Exodus 23:15a celebrates the Feast of Unleavened Bread (NIV)
- Exodus 23:16a celebrates the Feast of Harvest (NIV)
- Numbers 29:12a celebrates a festival to the *Lord* for seven days (NIV)
- Deuteronomy 16:13a celebrates the Feast of Tabernacles for seven days (NIV)
- Exodus 34:22a celebrates the Feast of Weeks (NIV)
- Numbers 9:4–5: "So Moses told the Israelites to celebrate the Passover" (NIV)
- Nehemiah 12:27: "At the dedication of the wall of Jerusalem, the Levites were sought out from where they lived and were brought to Jerusalem

to celebrate joyfully the dedication with songs of thanksgiving and with the music of cymbals, harps and lyres" (NIV).
- Luke 15:24: "For this son of mine was dead and is alive again; he was lost and is found. So they began to celebrate" (NIV).

In Genesis 2, we read that God walked with Adam and Eve in the Garden of Eden in the cool of the day. Adam and Eve fellowshipped and spoke with God on a regular basis. They were given chores to do in the Garden of Eden; they worked and took care of the plants and all the vegetation. Adam was given the privilege of naming all of the beasts of the earth, the birds, animals, and all livestock. So just sitting around and being idle is not what heaven is all about. There will be new and awesome things for us to do; we just won't know what they will be until we get there.

But for sure we will

- Worship
- Sing
- Dance
- Laugh
- Celebrate
- Play
- Help
- Rest
- Fellowship

- Talk with God
- Walk with God
- Learn
- Love

Worship and sing is kind of a scary thing for those of us who are pretty bad at it. But worshiping and singing will be a natural joy for us. The music will be wonderful and the best that we have ever heard or enjoyed before. Heaven will be the most exhilarating place in every aspect for us to live.

> Sing to the LORD a new song; sing to the LORD, all the earth. (Psalms 96:1, NIV)

> Sing and make music in your heart to the Lord. (Ephesians 5:19b, NIV)

> I will praise you, O Lord my God, with all my heart; I will glorify your name forever. For great is your love toward me; you have delivered me from the depths of the grave. (Psalm 86:12–13, NIV)

> Blessed are all who fear the LORD, who walk in his ways. (Psalms 128:1, NIV)

> Sing for joy, O heavens, for the LORD has done this; shout aloud, O earth beneath. Burst into song, you mountains, you forests and all your trees. (Isaiah 44:23, NIV)

We shall be entirely freed from the sufferings and adversities that we face in this life. Our future will involve a boundless, immeasurable, and never-ending genuine happiness in our new eternal home.

> But only the redeemed will walk there and the ransomed of the LORD will return. They will enter Zion with singing; everlasting joy will crown their heads. Gladness and joy will overtake them, and sorrow and sighing will flee away. (Isaiah 35:9–10, NIV)

When I Die Will I Be There Immediately, or Will I Have to Find a Certain Place?

Do not let your hearts be troubled. Trust in God; trust also in me. In my Father's house are many rooms; if it were not so, I would have told you. I am going there to prepare a place for you. And if I go and prepare a place for you, I will come back and take you to be with me that you also may be where I am. (John 14:1–3, NIV)

Will I need to find a trail or a light to find my way to heaven's gate? What if I can't find the right path? The thought of having to find our way on our own to enter heaven is extremely terrifying to say the least. My dad struggled with these questions. He was afraid that he wouldn't be able to find the right path or see a light in a tunnel to get to heaven. God has given us promises throughout scriptures that tell us that the blessed will see God face-to-face. This vision will be immediate and direct once our last breath on earth stops. We will find ourselves standing before our Savior Jesus at death. We will not have to find a path, a walkway, a light, or anything else to find our way to God. The Bible tells us that away from the body, at home with Lord. Immediately we will wake up in heaven; what a wonderful vow God has given us. He has promised us that we will be with Him wherever he is so that we don't have to worry about how to get to Him, He will come to us. Imagine God standing right next to you waiting to usher you into glory with him. Amen.

> Surely goodness and love will follow me all the days of my life and I will dwell in the house of the Lord forever. (Psalms 23:6, NIV)

> One thing I ask of the Lord, this is what I seek: that I may dwell in the house of the Lord all the days of my life. (Psalms 27:4, NIV)

> All honor to God, the God and Father of our Lord Jesus Christ; for it is his boundless mercy that has given us the privilege of being born again so that we are now members of God's own family. Now we live in the hope of eternal life because Christ rose again from the dead. And God has reserved for his children the priceless gift of eternal life; it is kept in heaven for you, pure and undefiled, beyond the reach of change and decay. And God, in his mighty power, will make sure that you get there safely to receive it because you are trusting him. It will be yours in that coming last day for all to see. So be truly glad! There is wonderful joy ahead, even though the going is rough for a while down here. (1 Peter 1:3–6, TLB)

I'm Afraid of Dying

When the perishable has been clothed with the imperishable and the mortal with immortality, then the saying that is written will come true: "Death has been swallowed up in victory." (1 Corinthians 15:54, NIV)

How is death swallowed up in victory? The sting of death is the thought that death has finality to it, it's the end all. Some think that when we die there's nothing else, it's the end of us completely. We are often led to believe this lie. God, on the other hand, says that death is not the ultimate end of our being but just the beginning of a great, exciting new journey. There is "victory" over death with the promise of heaven. Death is just the ending of the life we now live; there is so much more for those who love Christ. God has in store for us a brand-new journey that will be wildly amazing and will last forever. Death is our last enemy, but it will itself be destroyed and gone forever when we enter heaven's gate.

Who shall separate us from the love of Christ? For I am convinced that neither death nor life, neither angels nor demons, neither the present nor the future, nor any powers, neither height nor depth, nor anything else in all creation, will be able to

separate us from the love of God that is in Christ
Jesus our Lord. (Romans 8:35, 38–39, NIV)

MOST PEOPLE ARE AFRAID OF DYING

Death is an enemy, and we instinctively fear it with every
inch of our being. No one wants to contemplate about
dying; it's scary, frightening, and really morbid. Death in
all its ugliness is very factual and is something that we will
be confronted with eventually and have to face personally.
Death is an intruder that takes us by surprise even though
in the back of our minds we know that it is a real possibility.
Nobody wants to die; we all want to live forever. We don't
want to miss anything here on earth no matter how good
heaven sounds or how it is described.

Issues surrounding death and dying are not easy to talk
about since we live in a death-denying culture. Yet we live
in the shadow of death every single day; we just don't allow
ourselves to consider or think about it. Contemplating
death creates an enormous amount of anxiety for most of
us. It is very natural that people struggle with the thought
of transitioning from death to the hereafter. The thought of
never getting to see our loved ones again is overwhelmingly
heartbreaking. It seems so empty, so sad, so alone, and so
final. But it is not our final fate, it's just our relocation and
the beginning of something so amazing that there is no
way to describe what lies ahead for us.

The Bible is often viewed as a manuscript of death but
is truly a book of life. It actually proclaims the wonderful

power of a living God, the Creator of heaven and earth, whose authority has no boundaries or limitations. Because of the resurrection of Christ, our life after death is now a reality not just a hope. In His resurrection, Jesus conquered death—physically, spiritually, and eternally for all time.

God says repeatedly in the Bible that earth is our temporary home; we are just passing through. He also tells us not to get too comfortable with the things here and don't get so caught up in storing treasures here on earth. Our treasure, God reminds us over and over again, is in our next life with him. Everything that we collect or deem valuable today will not go with us; it will all stay behind. There was a bumper sticker several years ago that read something like this, "The one who dies with the most toys wins." And sometimes we get so engrossed in just that, collecting valuables, "stuff." What's prized here on earth is not prized in heaven; in fact, it carries no value at all. What God considers to be of the highest worth is *you and I. We* are priceless to God; it's not the things that we accumulate. So we are to live just one day at time while here on earth. Our permanent home is after we leave this earth and enter heaven's door.

> The Lord says, "Whoever loves me, I will save. I will protect those who know me. They will call to me, and I will answer them. I will be with them in trouble; I will rescue them and honor them." (Psalms 91:14–15, NIV)

God wants us to be absolutely sure of our destiny. He wants us to know positively that we are destined for eternity with him. We cling to the promise that God is holding out his hands and anxiously awaiting for us to show up in his heavenly home. Death can be peaceful for those who are dying and for those who love them and who stand by their side. Christ wants us to trust Him in both our living and our dying, letting Him comfort us through every aspect of our life.

> So do not fear, for I am with you; do not be dismayed, for I am your God. I will strengthen you and help you; I will uphold you with my righteous right hand. (Isaiah 41:10, NIV)

WORDS OF REASSURANCE AND PROMISE

About a week before my dad passed away, he said to me, "Pam, Jesus is real. He is standing right next to me. He has told me that I will be with him in just a few days." How comforting those words were for me and my dad. Those words will forever be etched in my memory. Christ revealed himself to my dad to comfort him and to take away all his fear. The fear of finding a tunnel or following a light was banished from my dad's thoughts completely. Calmness and comfort replaced the fear and anxiety that he had been fighting. How gracious was Christ to show himself to my dad to reassure him that he was there right next to his bedside. He passed away very peacefully a few days later, leaving this world for his next great adventure: heaven!

> For as high as the heavens are above the earth, so great is his love for those who fear him. (Psalms 103:11, NIV)

> We live by faith, not by sight. We are confident, I say, and would prefer to be away from the body and at home with the Lord. (2 Corinthians 5:7–8, NIV)

> To him who is able to keep you from falling and to present you before his glorious presence without fault and with great joy—to the only God our Savior be glory, majesty, power and authority, through Jesus Christ our Lord, before all ages, now and forevermore! Amen. (Jude 24, NIV)

> I write these things to you who believe in the name of the Son of God so that you may know that you have eternal life. (1 John 5:13, NIV)

WE HAVE AN INHERITANCE IN HEAVEN

God has promised us that in heaven we will receive an inheritance that will be

1. Safe
    - Free from harm, injury, not threatened by danger. We will be secure. Pain or destruction will never come to us again

2. Protected
    - We are kept safe, defended, and shielded from all evil forever.

3. Secure
    - We will never doubt that God is all powerful. We will be free of distrust, anxiety, or fear.

4. Glorious
    - We will praise, worship, and sing to God. God's all-brilliant glory will shine for eternity, wiping away any and all darkness. We will never see a shadow or anything frightening again. Great honor and praise we will give to the Lord

5. Magnificent
    - Heaven is the most stately, grandiose, lavish place. We are God's priceless creation, and He has a reserved a place for us to be with him.

6. Abundant
    - Our new home is abounding with generosity; there will be no "want" or "desire" for anything ever again.

7. Permanent
    - Never will we die again or be thrown out of heaven.

8. Everlasting
    - Our home forever, indefinitely and enduring through all of time.

9. Unending
    - Our new bodies will be ceaseless, dateless, and immortal

10. Loving
    - Abba Father, we have been adopted into God's family. God cherishes us totally and completely.

11. Priceless
    - We are God's treasure. The most highly valued thing in all of heaven by God.

The Lord will rescue me from every evil attack and will bring me safely to his heavenly kingdom. To him be glory forever and ever. Amen. (2 Timothy 4:18, NIV)

Praise be to the God and Father of our Lord Jesus Christ! In his great mercy he has given us new birth into a living hope through the resurrection of Jesus Christ from the dead, and into an inheritance that can never perish, spoil or fade kept in heaven for you. (1 Peter 1:3–4, NIV)

How Can I Be Certain That Heaven Will Be My Eternal Home?

This is the most crucial question anyone can ask. The answer has already been given; it's free, no strings attached. Knowing God is the single most important thing in your life. After all, we all want our names written in the book of life. It's not how much money we have or how much material wealth we have accumulated. What is most imperative is knowing for certain that our eternal life will be spent with God in heaven.

> Let him who is thirsty come; let him who desires take the water of life without price. (Revelations 22:1, NIV)

One day each of us will stand personally before God. God will then recount our life, and He will ask the most essential question in your life, "What did you do about Jesus?" He doesn't care about how many times you went to church or how much money you donated to worthy causes. He just wants to know if you said yes to Christ. The book of Romans tells us that if we confess with our mouth and believe in our heart that Jesus is Lord, we will be saved. We will forever live with Christ in his eternal home; God wants you to be sure without a doubt that heaven is your destiny. *Faith is the act of taking and accepting God's free gift of love and hope.*

> Therefore God exalted him to the highest place and gave him the name that is above every name, that at the name of Jesus every knee should bow, in heaven and on earth and under the earth, and every tongue confess that Jesus Christ is Lord, to the glory of God the Father. (Philippians 2:9–11, NIV)

God loves you so much that he collects your tears and knows the number of hairs on your head. What an awesome example of God's love for us. Our tears are so important that each of them is gathered together and then recorded in God's personal diary. The number of hairs on our head! How many hairs can that be collectively from all the people who love Christ? This seems like an unimaginable and unattainable task. Who else but God would even care about such things? Yet God knows all things, everything.

> You have seen me tossing and turning through the night. You have collected all my tears and preserved them in your bottle! You have recorded every one in your book. (Psalms 56:8, TLB)

> And even the very hairs of your head are all numbered. (Matthew 10:30, NIV)

It's by far the most important question for each of us to address. God wants you to know for certain that heaven waits for you.

> Here I am! I stand at the door and knock. If anyone hears my voice and opens the door, I will come in and eat with him, and he with me. (Revelation 3:20, NIV)

Christ stands outside the door of your heart and knocks softly, waiting patiently for you to open it. This door that he is standing in front of has no doorknob on his side. The doorknob is only on the other side, your side of the door. The only way for God to enter into your life is for you to turn the knob and open the door. Once you open that door and ask God for help and forgiveness, your name is written down in His book of life. He will never leave you, ever. He will help you through every single circumstance in your life. When a person says, "God, please forgive me and help me walk with you," the angels in heaven rejoice. God paints a fabulous picture for us, the angels singing, dancing, and celebrating that another person's future is now secured in heaven. You are now a child of the King forevermore, and heaven is your destination at death. God will be there when you close your eyes for the last time here on earth; He will be holding out his hands to you to welcome you to your new eternal home, heaven.

I tell you that in the same way there will be more rejoicing in heaven over one sinner who repents than over ninety-nine righteous persons who do not need to repent. (Luke 15:7, NIV)

I lift up my eyes to the hills where does my help come from? My help comes from the LORD, the Maker of heaven and earth. (Psalms 121:1–2, NIV)

I love those who love me and those who seek me find me. (Proverbs 8:17, NIV)

Seek the LORD while he may be found; call on him while he is near. (Isaiah 55:6, NIV)

"You will seek me and find me when you seek me with all your heart. I will be found by you," declares the LORD. (Jeremiah 29:13–14a, NIV)

Everyone who calls on the name of the Lord will be saved. (Romans 10:13, NIV)

When my children were young, I used to tell them all the time, "Don't try to grow up too fast. You're only a child for eighteen short years. You will be an adult a lot longer than being a child, so enjoy being a child." That too goes for us as to life here on earth. Our human body is temporary and not meant to live without end, but our new eternal body will be imperishable and designed to live forever. So in contrast to our life on earth, which is very short, eternity is for always and beyond the measure of time.

WHAT ABOUT CREMATION?

Many people today are contemplating cremation versus the normal burial with a casket. There are several factors why people are considering cremation today; a casket burial is costly, it takes a lot time and planning, it's faster and easier for loved ones left behind, and concern for land use is becoming highly important.

One reason that inground burial has been preferred by many is because the Bible teaches that one day those who die in Christ will be raised from the dead. But remember that God created us in the beginning, so God is able to bring back together whatever has been scattered, decayed, or torn apart. A body that has been destroyed by fire or any other circumstance will not prevent a sovereign God from resurrecting it to newness of life.

All bodies that are buried in a casket will go through the natural decomposing process. The cremation method rapidly speeds the decaying procedure along. Our heavenly body will be a completely new spiritual body. It will be nothing like our old bodies we have now that is made of flesh and blood.

> It is the same with the dead who are raised to life.
> The body that is "planted" will ruin and decay, but
> it is raised to a life that cannot be destroyed. When

the body is "planted," it is without honor, but it is raised in glory. When the body is "planted," it is weak, but when it is raised, it is powerful. The body that is "planted" is a physical body. When it is raised, it is a spiritual body. (1 Corinthians 15:42–44, NCV)

When this happens when our perishable earthly bodies have been transformed into heavenly bodies that will never die then at last the Scriptures will come true: "Death is swallowed up in victory. O death, where is your victory? O death, where is your sting?" For sin is the sting that results in death, and the law gives sin its power. How we thank God, who gives us victory over sin and death through Jesus Christ our Lord! (1 Corinthians 15:54–57, NLT)

Whatever method of final disposition a person chooses for burial should be arranged with dignity and honor. Remember to keep in mind that your family's needs for closure are extremely important. Some family members may not be able to cope with the cremation process. So an intimate discussion on how a person is to be buried is advantageous for everyone involved prior to the actual event.

REVELATION 21:1–8 (NIV)

Then I saw a new heaven and a new earth, for the first heaven and the first earth had passed away, and there was no longer any sea. I saw the holy city, the New Jerusalem, coming down out of heaven from God, prepared as a bride beautifully dressed for her husband. And I heard a loud voice from the throne saying, "Now the dwelling of God is with men, and he will live with them. They will be his people, and God himself will be with them and be their God. He will wipe every tear from their eyes. There will be no more death or mourning or crying or pain, for the old order of things has passed away."

He who was seated on the throne said, "I am making everything new!" Then he said, "Write this down, for these words are trustworthy and true."

He said to me: "It is done. I am the Alpha and the Omega, the Beginning and the End. To him who is thirsty I will give to drink without cost from the spring of the water of life. He who overcomes will inherit all this, and I will be his God and he will be my son. But the cowardly, the unbelieving, the vile, the murderers, the sexually immoral, those who practice magic arts, the idolaters and all liars — their place will be in the fiery lake of burning sulfur. This is the second death."

PSALMS 100

A psalm for giving thanks.

Shout for joy to the LORD, all the earth.
Worship the LORD with gladness ;
come before him with joyful songs.
Know that the LORD is God.
It is he who made us, and we are his;
we are his people, the sheep of his pasture.
Enter his gates with thanksgiving
and his courts with praise;
give thanks to him and praise his name.
For the LORD is good and his love endures forever;
his faithfulness continues through all generations.
(NIV Translation)